The Addictive Personal Trainer

The Client-Centered Training Approach

That KeepsThem Coming Back for More!

Rhonda K. Huff
M.ED, AADP, CPT, CHHC

The Addictive Personal Trainer

The Client-Centered Training Approach
That Keeps Them Coming Back for More!

Rhonda K. Huff

M.ED, AADP, CPT, CHHC

A Glowing Swan Publication

The Addictive Personal Trainer
The Client-Centered Training Approach
That Keeps Them Coming Back for More!

ISBN 978-1-938579-17-2

10 9 8 7 6 5 4 3 2 1

Cover design by Bobbi Parker
Author photo by Bobbi Parker Photography
Editing and design by Karen Morgan

A Glowing Swan Publication
New York, Virginia

Printed in the United States of America

Dedications

To my mom, Kay Norman Huff: You raised me to believe there was nothing I couldn't do if I set my mind to it. That resolve has served me well throughout life, especially during my battle with breast cancer.

To my high school English teacher, Mr. Phillip Parrish: You took the time to teach a terrified teenager how to speak confidently in public. I know I wouldn't be where I am today without your patient and sacrificial guidance.

To my very best friend, Sheila Zych: You have never ever ever stopped believing in me, loving me, encouraging me and pushing me to be the best I can be and to never settle for less! God put you in my life when I needed an angel, and I'm so glad he chose you!

Contents

Acknowledgments xi

Introduction 1

Chapter 1: Get the ball rolling 3

Tip One: Set goals 4
Tip Two: Face your fears 7
Tip Three: Get personal and professional referrals 9
Tip Four: Get testimonials 11
Tip Five: Network 12

Chapter 2: What the Client Wants 13

Tip One: Listen to what the client is saying 14
Tip Two: Listen to what the client is NOT saying 17
Tip Three: Help clients set goals 19
Tip Four: Help clients determine their challenges 21
Tip Five: Help prepare them to conquer challenges ... 23

Chapter 3: What the Client Needs........................ 25

Tip One: Discover wants versus needs 26
Tip Two: Choose the right assessments 28
Tip Three: Determine imbalances and deficits............30
Tip Four: Discover Primary Food™ needs 33
Tip Five: Determine commitment...............................35

Chapter 4: The "Eyes" Have It............................ 38

Tip One: Understand that this is not your workout.....39
Tip Two: Communicate..40
Tip Three: Demonstrate 42
Tip Four: Coach 43
Tip Five: Evaluate 45

Chapter 5: Attention!... 46

Tip One: Greet them with excitement.........................47
Tip Two: Take good notes...49
Tip Three: Eliminate distractions 50
Tip Four: Ask about their day/week...........................52
Tip Five: Let them know that you enjoy them............54

Chapter 6: Trust Me!... 56

Tip One: Keep what is said in private, private............57
Tip Two: Do what you say you will do.......................58
Tip Three: Offer accountability..................................59

Tip Four: Be strong..61
Tip Five: Be real — not the stereotypical trainer........63

Chapter 7: Encourage, encourage, encourage........... 66

Tip One: Realize everyone needs encouragement 67
Tip Two: Make the client want to be around you.......69
Tip Three: Celebrate the small victories....................71
Tip Four: Laugh A LOT..72
Tip Five: Help them be positive..................................74

Chapter 8: Learn More, Earn More 76

Tip One: Stay up to date on research and trends.........77
Tip Two: Become the go-to expert..............................79
Tip Three: Learn about nutrition 80
Tip Four: Learn life/health coaching 85
Tip Five: Surround yourself with experts...................86

Appendix...93

About the Author 95

What People are Saying...97

Acknowledgments

There are so many people who have given me the encouragement I needed to write this book. My editor, Karen Morgan, (also the Features Editor of the Daily Press) kept sending me things written by other fitness professionals and saying "You need to do this!" She, along with Karen Kashtan, finally convinced me that I had something to say.

A word of prophesy was spoken over me almost exactly a year ago at Beauty for Ashes Ministry in Newport News, VA. The evangelist said to me "You write…but you write for yourself. God wants you to write for others." Wow! Who would've known!

My "kids," Matt and Andi Greene, Ashtyn Greene, Zack Villanueva-Smith, Trey, Chaysen, and Kayde Brooks are a constant source of encouragement to me every single day of my life! Everything I do, I do with them in mind!

Drew and Karin Rozell taught me so much about how to be an entrepreneur, not just an author. The process of putting together a book from start to finish and having total control of it all has been exhilarating!

Bill and Mary Linda Carmines took me under their wing, literally, when I needed it most.

My dad, Bill Huff and my sister and brother-in-law, Michele and Steve Brooks, are sweet constants in my life.

A few of my awesome interns — Karen, Tirza, Kat, Andi, and Teresa — gave me feedback on the first draft.

My clients, who are the most inspiring people I know. I have learned more from them than any textbook! Working with them gave me the knowledge and insight for this book.

And basically everyone else in my life! I love you and am thankful for you!

Introduction

I had a client tell me that people were addicted to me and couldn't stand to miss a workout session with me. Although the statement made me laugh, I decided to explore the implications of that comment. As I started talking to my clients about why they continued training with me, I saw a pattern develop. That pattern led to this book.

Many of my clients were formerly trained by a typical trainer at a local gym. They said they felt the trainer was just going through the motions and totally uninterested in their progress, much less their life. They sometimes felt the trainer was pushing them harder than they wanted to be pushed (although I submit that when encouraged properly by a trusted trainer, those tougher limits become welcomed). They often said they felt worse about themselves after hiring the trainer. They wanted someone to encourage them and make them feel good about themselves.

When you give them that, they keep coming back. That feeling of confidence is addictive!

My secret weapon is simple, yet effective, and my clients stay satisfied and continue to come back for more. Not only do they enjoy the health benefits of lower blood pressures, improved blood lipid profiles, better lean body mass percentages, improved bone density ratios, and decreased pain; they also improve their confidence levels, their outlook on life, their ability to laugh at themselves and others, their relationships with others, and their relationship with food.

That feeling of empowerment is addictive!

I gain clients solely through word of mouth advertising. These referrals come from existing clients and medical referrals. My first year in business turned a profit. That almost never happens. It usually takes at least five years to create a profitable business, but I did it the first year, and you can, too! Just follow the simple guidelines in this book and become your clients' best addiction!

Chapter 1:
Get the ball rolling

"You don't have to be great to get started, but you have to get started to be great."

Les Brown

Tip One:
Set goals

You have gotten the proper education and certification —
so what now? Peter Drucker, a self-described "social ecologist"
taught that "the best way to predict the future is to create it."
What are you doing to create your personal training career?
Don't think you can just sit back and wait for clients to find you!
Your perfect client may not even know he or she needs you!

What motivates you? Making a name for yourself? Helping
your community? Making enough money to move out of your
parents' house? Having some fun money to do some traveling?
Write down why you want a personal training career. If you
aren't sure, do some journaling about what you are feeling and
discuss it with a friend or family member. Determine what is
blocking the motivational flow.

Once you have determined what motivates you, set some
goals around that motivation. You may actually discover that
your motivation changes as you begin to set goals and that
is okay. It is a process — trust the process and embrace what
comes from it. Follow the secret of improv comedians — always
say "yes." This can be hard to do, but it is not impossible. It
takes a mind shift. Instead of resisting the things happening in
your life, discover the possibilities that may be there just waiting
to bring you success.

I like to set long-, medium-, and short–term goals.

I begin with my long-term (I use 10 years) goals and then
move to my medium-term (five years) and short-term (one year)
goals.

I use this order so that my one- and five-year goals are in-line with and supportive of my ultimate 10-year goals.

If your long-term goal is to own an athletic training center, why would you make a one-year goal of working in a gym that only trains the general population? Seek out opportunities with people who are already doing what you ultimately want to do. You will grow your knowledge, experience, and contacts all at the same time. Plus, it will either reinforce your direction or it will cause you to rethink it.

Next, set your financial goals.

List your personal expenses (include fun money!):

List your business expenses:

How much do you want to save or invest per month?

How much do you want to give away each month?

Add up all of your expenses. This is how much you need to make each month.

Multiply by 12. This is your needed yearly income.

Now determine how many clients you need to make this happen and get busy!

Tip Two:
Face your fears

I have heard it all. And truth be told, I have felt it all too. The enemy knows how to get me stuck. Just place a little fear — sometimes disguised as doubt — into my mind. Let's get a few of these thoughts on — or should I say OFF — the table.

I don't know enough.
Yes you do. And you will learn more and more every time you work with someone.

I'm afraid of rejection.
We all are. Do it anyway. There really is no such thing as rejection, only selection. So what if they don't choose you, someone else will.

I don't know how to get started.
Then ask someone. Or at least Google it.

I'm not as good as so and so.
And they think they are not as good as someone else. We all have our strengths and weaknesses. Embrace your strengths, work on your weaknesses, and keep moving forward.

What if my clients don't think I am perfect enough?
They don't expect you to be perfect. They expect you to be real and to support them. It's about them, not you.

What if my clients don't reach their goals?

Ultimately it is their responsibility. You are there to guide and encourage. If they see you three hours per week, they have 165 hours to mess it up.

I am afraid of success.

Yes. This is a very real fear. Ask yourself, "If I succeed, what will it mean? Will I have less time for family? Will I have less time to enjoy other hobbies? Will people expect too much of me? Will people treat me differently? Will I lose my old friends?" Explore this possible fear because it is often overlooked.

Don't allow fear to keep you stuck. You are amazing. You know enough.

You can help so many people. Now go find them!

Tip Three:
Get personal
and professional referrals

If you are just starting out and still waiting for client No.1, don't be afraid to ask people you know for referrals. Most people are happy to help and enjoy feeling like they contributed to your success. Remember to thank them with a card or a small token gift. They won't expect much; they know you are just starting out.

I have also met people in Starbucks, the grocery store, and other public places who have become clients. This is easier for those of you who are more extroverted. People are always talking about their health. Just keep your ears tuned in and give them a smile and your business card. Before you know it, they will be addicted to you, too.

A happy client is absolutely the best way to get new clients. The very nature of personal training is "PERSONAL." People looking for someone to help them on a journey as intimate as their health, appreciate knowing that someone already trusts you and has experienced success with you. When clients meet a goal, celebrate the goal and ask them if your services helped them reach that goal. When they emphatically shout "YES" ask them if they know anyone else who could use your services. Don't feel awkward about asking. If they are happy about how you have helped them, they will want to return the favor.

Offer incentives. I offer one free session if their referral signs up for a full month of training. But you can be as creative as you want. Create something that your clients will want to work toward. Have competitions. Have your clients "team-up" with a new referral and whoever wins the competition gets something special. I once gave trophies and my clients loved it. One guy said it was the first thing he had ever won. It was really fun, my clients got to know each other, and it cost me very little.

Professional referrals are also a great way to get clients. Build trusting relationships with medical professionals in your area. These can be doctors, nurses, naturopaths, chiropractors, physical therapists, dieticians, and fitness professionals that offer complementary services to yours such as yoga or pilates instructors. Remember to return the favor and refer people to them as well.

Tip Four:
Get testimonials

I was too embarrassed to ask for testimonials for the longest time. Finally someone who knows a lot more than I do about marketing said my website needed testimonials. So I worked up the courage to finally ask a few people whom I knew wouldn't say no. Their testimonials were amazing. It was such an encouragement to me to know the positive impact that they felt I had placed on their lives, not just on their health. It made me feel a totally different type of empowered confidence in what I am doing.

I have a section on my website just for testimonials, but I haven't placed many on there yet because it still embarrasses me a bit. One thing is certain, though, when I get the website analytics each month, the testimonial page is the most viewed page. Testimonials will not only make your potential clients feel confident about trusting you with their health but they will lift you up and give you the encouragement to keep moving forward with your purpose.

Tip Five:
Network

According to Merriam-Webster, networking is simply "the exchange of information or services among individuals, groups, or institutions." There are so many ways to network these days. Social networking such as Facebook, Twitter, blogs, and websites can help you get your message to the public. Networking groups such as Business Networking International (BNI), and others like them, get you in front of people who become your marketing network by spreading the word about you (in exchange for you doing the same for them). The Chamber of Commerce also works on behalf of local businesses by advocating for them within the community. Other ways to network include giving lectures or workshops, sending out newsletters, attending cultural or sporting events, participating in trade shows or health fairs, and donating services to charity events.

Do your research before jumping into any of these. It is imperative that you target audiences that fall within your niche. Otherwise, you could be wasting a lot of time, money, and effort.

If you choose live networking events, be professional. These events should be looked upon as a business venture, not a social one. Listen more than you talk (ask open-ended questions). Make appropriate eye contact. Be pleasant, not pushy. Mingle and meet new people — step out of your comfort zone. Have your business cards handy and offer something to the people you meet. Eat before you go. Stay focused on building professional relationships.

Chapter 2:
What the Client Wants

"I remind myself every morning:
Nothing I say this day will teach me
anything. So if I'm going to learn,
I must do it by listening."

Larry Kin

Tip One:
Listen to what the client is saying

Michael J. Marquardt, professor of human resources and international affairs at George Washington University and author of *Leading with Questions: How Leaders Find the Right Solutions by Knowing What to Ask*, says that when you ask empowering questions you convey respect for the person and actually encourage that person's development as a thinker and problem solver. This serves two purposes in your personal training business. It gives the client the short-term value of generating a solution to the issue at hand (their health) and also the long-term value of providing the tools to handle similar issues in the future.

Your clients already know what they should be doing to be healthy. They just need validation.

When taking their health histories ask them what three things they should be doing for their health but aren't.

Most people will very quickly give you two: exercise and eat better.

The third response will tell you the most about your clients. Make the third response your first objective and the other two will follow.

Help your clients think analytically and critically. When they tell you about their exercise and nutrition programs — or lack thereof — ask them what the consequences to their choices have been so far. Be understanding and never judge what they say. You want to be a vessel through which living water can pour into their lives. Whatever they tell you is OK. It's their personal realities. Move them from that to what the future could hold if they hire you to help them. Once again, allow them to produce the answers to their own dilemmas. You are just the guide.

You may need to challenge deeply rooted assumptions. If they have "tried every diet," "always been overweight," "are just big-boned," "tried lifting weights before but it didn't work" or any other lie that they have bought into, you will need to help them deconstruct where and why those beliefs began. This will be an ongoing process. We all know how hard it is to "turn off the recorder" in our own brains so be sympathetic and support-ive. However, do not let them wallow in it. Their results and your reputation depend on it.

Nurture communication by eliminating communication roadblocks. A roadblock is simply a situation that prevents prog-ress. Therefore, certain questions and intonations can stop the open communication you are seeking.

Possibly the most important thing is to eliminate the ques-tion "why?" from your sessions. When you follow a comment with the question "why?" it automatically makes you sound judgmental and puts clients on the defensive. A "why" forces people to answer with a "because" so they can justify their ac-tions. Therefore, the client feels they have to justify to you even though you were probably just trying to get more information. If you think this sounds far-fetched, try it out on your family and friends. Notice how the conversation changes and how the am-bience becomes tense. You can probably even remember times when someone has asked you "why?" and how you felt about explaining your decision to them. A better follow up would sim-ply be, "Tell be more about that."

Don't offer quick assurances, such as, "Don't worry about that." You may be trying to make things better for them but it sounds like you are making light of the situation. Just because you don't worry about certain things doesn't mean you have the right to tell someone else they shouldn't. This can stop a conversation cold.

Never patronize. Saying things like, "You poor thing" will not do anything to help them solve their problems. You want to provide clients with empowerment and confidence. Patronizing never yields those results.

Resist giving advice. There will be times when you feel an overwhelming urge to provide a solution. Don't! Remember, the goal is to empower clients so they can synthesize their own solutions. Comments that say either, "You should…" or "I think the best thing for you to do is…" completely steal their power from them.

While they are talking, be patient. Interrupting them can make them forget their line of thought or discourage them from continuing to discuss the situation. Also, silence should not be avoided. Sometimes a bit of silence once they have stopped talking will prompt them to go deeper. The deeper they go, the more progress they will make. However, never push clients to talk about things that make them uncomfortable. When the time is right, they will talk. Until then, offer support, encouragement, and hope. That is really what most people need anyway.

Tip Two:
Listen to what the client is NOT saying

Our eyes are our greatest source of knowledge.

Communication is approximately 55 percent body language, 38 percent voice/tone, and 7 percent words (isucceedbook.com)

You will learn a lot about your clients from observing their actions and hearing the underlying tones of what they are telling you.

Are they comfortable with you? This is obvious if their body posture is relaxed and they are leaning toward you. If they are leaning back and have their arms crossed, you need to change the atmosphere in the room.

Are there pauses or delays in their responses? Sometimes they are just thinking. Other times they are getting ready to lie to you. You may see this when you ask them how much they exercise or what they eat. Do they change the subject? That is OK. If it's a question that must be answered for the clients' safety, such as a medical question, come back to it later. They may just need to warm up to you. It can be hard sharing private information with a stranger. If they still resist, lovingly let them know you need the information to make sure you can design the best and safest program for them. Also inform them that the information is held in strict confidence, and then make sure you do that.

Are their answers vague? Do they look away when answering questions? Do they get defensive easily? All of these behaviors will help you get the big picture of what your clients are all about.

With practice, this unspoken information will allow you to

reach your clients when no one else may have been able to reach them. You will be able to discern if they need a sweet, caring, understanding trainer, a drill sergeant, or something in between. And when you demonstrate through your own responses that you really "get them," they will not walk away. You will have gained a client and your client will have gained a professional who can truly help him reach his goals. It's a win-win!

Tip Three:
Help clients set goals

All of your potential clients will come to you with goals. That is one of the reasons they have sought you out in the first place. They have probably tried to reach their goals on their own and failed. If you are S.M.A.R.T. about this, you can decipher why their goals have failed and help them set ones that are destined to succeed with your guidance.

S.M.A.R.T. is an acrostic used to set goals. Good goals are Specific, Measureable, Attainable, Realistic, and Timely. This tool helps people make definite decisions about the goals they want to meet.

However, if you are as busy as I am — or if you want to be eventually — you need things simple, concise, and quick. I juggle many jobs, and I like to keep them as streamlined as possible, so I suggest something much simpler. Fill in the blanks:

I will _____

(Example: Lose two dress sizes in three months, which is going to be approximately 20 pounds or just under 2 pounds per week)

By doing _____

(Example: Working with a personal trainer three times a week)

When_____

(Example: On Mondays, Wednesdays, and Fridays from 10-11 a.m.)

I will measure my progress by_____

(Example: Trying on my goal dress once per week to gauge progress. They should be down one dress size in six weeks to be on target.)

This chart is easy to understand and easy to modify. For instance if your client is working out three days per week but eating Twinkies for dinner every night, the measurement aspect will quickly show that something is amiss. At that point, you simply help your client make adjustments to the chart.

The end result is the CLIENT'S responsibility. Your responsibility is to guide, encourage, and offer insight.

Tip Four:
Help clients determine their challenges

Just as important as the goal itself is the knowledge that many factors can inhibit the attainment of that goal. Willpower alone is usually not enough to reach a goal. There are elusive forces behind a person's willpower that science is still trying to understand. Researchers are finding that willpower is a mental muscle, and many factors, physically and mentally, can strengthen or weaken this muscle.

Florida State University researchers showed a relationship between willpower and blood glucose levels and found that restoring glucose levels to an appropriate level led to an increase in willpower. This is important to you as a trainer because many of your clients will try fad diets that are essentially starvation-type diets that will cause their blood glucose levels to drop. Glucose fuels many brain functions and when they can't resist the chocolate cake, they feel like a failure, and will often stop trying. It is a vicious cycle. Get them off the diet merry-go-round!

Sometimes the most powerful challenges to a goal are the messages that get played over and over in our minds. These messages can be from a critical parent, a coach, a bully, or anyone else who had some form of control over the client. These messages can be buried deeply inside and cocooned to prevent further pain. As the client becomes more comfortable with you, it may become necessary to help them get victory over these negative messages. Once again, your job is support only. The client already has the answers. You are not teaching them anything. Never step outside your scope of practice and when in doubt, refer out!

When I ask for a client to set goals, I always have them to write down the challenges they feel they may face in trying to accomplish these goals. Usually it takes some good high-mileage questions to get to the real root of the challenge. But it is essential to their success. Don't skip this important step.

For each challenge, the client needs to have a solution. What is their escape route when this challenge raises its ugly head, which we know it will relentlessly? Resist the temptation to give them the answers you think will help. Your clients need to be in charge of their own results.

Tip Five:
Help prepare them to conquer challenges

Now that goals are set and challenges are identified, it is time to get started on some specific action steps. Most of the planning has already been done by now so all that is left is to help them put it into a reasonable to-do list. It will look something like this:

Goal No. 1:

"I will lose two dress sizes in three months"

Challenge: I am addicted to sugar

Solution: I will add sweet vegetables to my diet and eat something green before I eat anything else. If I want a candy bar, I will eat kale first!

By nourishing the body, the client will have less and less cravings for sugar. A craving for sugar is a cry for energy. Add energy-rich foods instead of taking away their addiction. The addiction will take care of itself if they do what you ask. And you will know.

"By working with a personal trainer three times per week."

Challenge: It is really expensive.

Solution: If I skip Starbucks and make my own coffee in

the mornings and take my lunch instead of ordering out, I can make it work.

*"On Mondays, Wednesdays, and Fridays
from 6-7 p.m."*

Challenge: I work full time and just want to go home at the end of my workday
Solution: No refund if I miss a workout.

*"I will measure my progress
by trying on my dress once a week."*
They should be down one size in six weeks to be on target.

*"I will reward myself by getting
a massage and a manicure."*
Do NOT allow the client to reward themselves with food.

Chapter 3:
What the Client Needs

"To listen fully means to pay close attention to what is being said beneath the words. You listen not only to the 'music' but to the essence of the person speaking. You listen not only for what someone knows, but for what he or she is..."

Peter Senge

Tip One:
Discover wants versus needs

People hire personal trainers for many different reasons. They may not be seeing results on their own, they may be bored with their current workout, they may not know where to begin, they may need accountability and motivation, they may be training for an athletic event, they may be recovering from an injury or illness, or they may want to lose weight, gain weight, tone up, or gain muscle mass.

As you complete your goal-setting session and begin your fitness evaluation, you may see some areas that must be addressed before they can safely reach their goals.

For example, a 25-year-old male wants to hire you to help him gain muscle mass. As you evaluate him, you notice he has horrible posture. Can you safely bulk him up without addressing posture? No! Therefore you must explain what the program would entail in order to get his joints and the stressed tendons and ligaments in shape before you can start adding heavy weight to his workout.

Perhaps the client has worked out for years but is no longer seeing results. She may have a certain type of program that she prefers and is reluctant to try something new. It is your job to determine what type of training style may help her get past her plateau.

Suppose a wife has come in at her husband's request to lose weight. She may be completely humiliated and hurt by this. She wants to lose weight (she thinks) but she may need unconditional support from you to restore her confidence and to help her understand the concept of self-care before she will invest the time in losing weight.

Someone coming to you fresh out of physical therapy may feel ready to get back to heavy lifting; but there may still be some significant strength or balance deficits that must be addressed first. The evaluation will show these deficits and allow you to explain to the client what you are seeing and how you can help.

Be patient with yourself here. As a new trainer, it may take some practice to get really good at the skill of determining a client's unspoken needs. Celebrate yourself each time you get it right! There is so much personal satisfaction gained by helping people and that will fuel you to keep striving to improve your skills as a trainer.

Tip Two:
Choose the right assessments

There are so many evaluation tools in this industry. Learn about them and determine the types of clients who would best benefit from them.

Would you do the YMCA 3-Minute Step Test on an older individual with poor balance? Of course not! Sometimes there will be people who cannot safely do any of the assessments. What do you do with those people? Be honest with them, but also be sensitive. You may explain that there are some assessments that you want to do as a future goal. Give them a time goal to get this done. And when they are able to perform the assessment, even if the result is poor, there still should be a little celebration!

I have worked with many clients who are absolutely scared to death to work out. They are convinced they will get hurt. When assessing these individuals, do not push if they are hesitant to try something. It is not that important. You simply start from the beginning with them. Also, make sure you give them something to do with which they will experience success each time they are with you. For example, I have a client who will struggle through balance moves, but if I put a ball in her hands — she is a former basketball player — she can do whatever I ask of her. Holding that ball makes her feel like a superstar. That feeling of victory is a tremendous motivator and will make your clients want to experience the feeling again. We are all sort of like Pavlov's dog!

I have heard some trainers almost berate potential clients to make them feel like they cannot survive without hiring them.

This approach almost never works and starts the trainer/client relationship out on unequal terms. Your clients need to feel you are their support system and are right there with them throughout the process.

Tip Three:
Determine imbalances and deficits

Positive health is associated with the ability to enjoy life and withstand challenges. Our bodies desire to be perfectly balanced. When we move, our muscles, tendons, and ligaments all help to move our skeleton. If there is an imbalance or deficit in even a single muscle, all the others have to make up for it and movement becomes compromised. Once movement is compromised, injuries are more likely to occur and the ability to enjoy life and withstand challenges will suffer.

Check their posture. Hang a plumb line from the ceiling (a long piece of yarn with a small bolt tied to the bottom works fine). Have the client face the plumb line. You will immediately see postural imbalances at the shoulders, hips, knees, and ankles. Also take note of how the hands lie by their sides. The palms should face their sides, not behind them. Then have them turn sideways. Now you will see if they have lordosis, kyphosis, rounded shoulders, or a forward head position (for every inch the head moves forward in posture, it increases the weight of the head on the neck by 10 pounds (www.necksolutions.com)) Also, make note of any muscles that are smaller on one side.

Check their balance. Even young people sometimes have balance problems. Have them stand on one leg with their hands on their hips and one foot placed alongside the opposite leg (keep pressure off the knee joint by allowing them to place the foot on the lower leg and instruct them to not push the foot into the leg). See if they can hold their balance without moving their hands or their foot for one minute. Balance training can be modified. If holding one foot up is too hard, have them take a wide base of support and close their eyes. (Believe it or not, some people cannot even do that.) Once the wide base of support is easy, have them put their feet together with the eyes closed. Eventually they will improve and once the one-leg stand is mastered, you can move to more advanced balance work.

Another important component of balance is proprioception, which is the body's ability to interpret and utilize information about your position in space. This information comes to us through cues from the bottom of the feet, the relation of the inner ear to gravity, and what the eyes see. Using this environmental feedback system, the body senses which muscles to activate and deactivate to maintain a specific position in space.

For clients with really bad balance, I begin by having them remove their shoes in order to have a better connection between their feet and the floor. I also encourage people to walk around barefoot as much as they can. The foot and ankle contain 26 bones (one-quarter of the bones in the human body are in the feet), 33 joints, more than 100 muscles, tendons and ligaments, and a network of blood vessels, nerves, skin, and soft tissue. These muscles need to be worked. Barefoot walking strengthens every muscle in your feet and lower legs. It will help your client regain proper function of the feet by strengthening the arches, reducing bunions, and straightening out the toes. And when your client's feet feel better, his whole body feels better and he will be addicted to you.

As they go through their workouts, you will want to monitor their body mechanics to determine if they have strength or flexibility deficits.

Do the extremities move through the proper range of motion or is the client favoring one side? Can the client lift the same amount of weight on each side with roughly the same effort? Does one side of the barbell reach the endpoint of the exercise before the other side? Does the client pull slightly to one side when doing abdominal work? Are the muscles more pronounced on one side of the body? Do lunges look the same on both sides or does the client lean forward on one side in order to drop as low as the other side? Observe and note.

By repairing strength and flexibility deficits, the client will notice a wonderful difference in doing activities of daily living. They will enjoy more energy, increased stamina, and a new level of confidence. You will be hailed as a miracle worker, and your client will be addicted.

I had a client who came to me so incredibly kyphotic that her doctor wanted her to consider using a wheelchair. She asked if I could help her. Although I really wasn't sure just by looking at her, I said "I will sure try!" Within four months, she was upright and enjoying many things that she hadn't been able to enjoy in a long time. Her doctor later called me and asked what I had done. My response was, "I strengthened a few muscles."

You have the knowledge and the power to help people love themselves and love life. That is a true gift, my friend!

Tip Four:
Discover Primary Food™ needs

There are primary foods and secondary foods. Surprisingly, secondary foods are the foods we eat. Primary foods are relationships, career, physical activity, and spirituality. If your client is fulfilled in her primary food, the food she eats will be in its rightful place — second. Clients who have unhealthy relationships with food are dissatisfied in at least one primary food. If you would like to learn more about Primary Foods™, a concept developed by Joshua Rosenthal, the founder of the Institute for Integrative Nutrition®, check out my website's homepage, www.rhondakhuff.com, for a free download of Joshua's book titled *Integrative Nutrition: Feed Your Hunger for Health and Happiness*. This is a fabulous resource to use with your clients.

It is fairly easy to determine the health of someone's primary foods. Most people love to talk about themselves and just want to be heard. Even doctors are too busy to really listen anymore so you may be the first person in a long time who has actually listened to this person.

Remember to ask high-mileage questions, not ones that can be answered with a yes or no. By simply saying, "Tell me more about that." or asking "How does that make you feel?" you will begin to discern what things are going well or not so well for your client. As your relationship with your client deepens, you will be able to help her talk through many things that have led to where she is right now.

You may be thinking, "I can't do this. I'm not a counselor." You are right! YOU can't do it! But the client can...and with your support, will. We all know what we need; we just have to hear ourselves speak it. Once again — and you will hear me say this several times in the book — remember your scope of practice and when in doubt, refer out.

Tip Five:
Determine commitment

The American College of Sports Medicine (ACSM) guidelines are divided into three categories for cardiorespiratory fitness (CRF). In other words, this doesn't even include time for resistance training, yoga, pilates, or other health-related exercise goals.

Category	Frequency	Intensity	Time	Equivalent to:
Avoidance of disease	5 days per week	Moderate	30 min.	Walking 6-12 miles per week
Fitness	3-4 days per week	Vigorous	30-45 min.	Jogging 10 miles per week
Performance	7 days per week	Very vigorous	2 hours per day	Running 100 miles per week

Now, let's look at what ACSM says about strength training...

Do 8-10 exercises for the major muscle groups: legs, hips, back, chest, shoulders, biceps, triceps (core is missing from their chart)	To maximize strength development, use a resistance that allows 8-12 reps of each exercise, resulting in muscle fatigue	One set of each exercise is sufficient, but more can be gained with 2 or 3 sets.	Do resistance training on 2 or more nonconsecutive days each week.

Some observations:

1. Using a standard cadence, this would result in approximately 20 minutes — 4+ hours per week.

2. Add in the above recommended cardio for the Avoidance of Disease and Fitness Categories only and you have 2 — 6.25+ hours per week of exercise.

3. Suppose they want to participate in a yoga or meditation class for stress reduction? Add that time into their schedule as well.

4. And keep in mind: Exercise that extends beyond 60 minutes at a time in populations that are at risk

for disease, increases cortisol, which may decrease bone density, suppress the immune system, increase vascular constriction, and decrease insulin sensitivity. (*International Journal of Endocrinology and Metabolism;" Exercise and the Stress System*; 2005)

So, the clients who want to be regulars at your gym and are not at risk for disease, great! Get them started and monitor their progress. It will be very important for you to keep them motivated. It is hard to stay motivated at these levels unless you are a die-hard exerciser. So the question becomes, how much exercise can they regularly maintain without getting bored, frustrated, or injured? The industry cannot tell you this; only your clients can. So, listen carefully to what they are saying and not saying about their time and lifestyle.

However, to prescribe a busy and stressed-out female executive 30 minutes of cardio most days of the week and 2-3 days of hour-long strength training is a recipe for failure. How long do you think she will physically and mentally be able to comply? It will be almost impossible. She may need to train on fewer days, in less time, and with higher (much higher) intensity. This form of exercise is characterized by a high level of effort in a short period of time — between 10 and 30 minutes per workout. Nautilus inventor Arthur Jones helped define and popularize high intensity training in the 1970s, often summarizing the general philosophy as "...train harder, but train less often."

The bottom line is simply that you must be a student of your client. Each person will respond a little differently to the demands of exercise — physically, mentally, emotionally, spiritually, and socially. If you can put all the pieces together in a way that gives your clients success and satisfaction, they will stay with you forever. You will become their healthy addiction.

Chapter 4:
The "Eyes" Have It

"The moment one gives close
attention to anything, even a
blade of grass, it becomes a
mysterious, awesome,
indescribably magnificent
world in itself."

Henry Miller

Tip One:
Understand that this
is not your workout

I take great issue with trainers who claim they work out with their clients in order to better motivate them. If you are not watching — or in some cases, touching — your clients, you do not know what is going on with their workouts. Is their form perfect? Do they have a strength, size, or balance deficit on one side? Where are they "pushing" through the exercise instead of steadily "flowing" through it? What happens if they need your help? What happens if they get injured and you didn't see what happened?

My clients know I am there for them 100 percent. If they get into trouble, I am there to rescue them. If they get the form wrong, I am there to correct it. They pay me to train them; not to get my own workout.

Tip Two:
Communicate

People learn through hearing (auditory), seeing (visual), and doing (kinetic). The learning curve improves greatly when someone is exposed to all three learning styles. Our field naturally allows for this.

Your clients will be using the auditory learning style when you verbally communicate the exercise to them.

This is the "what" and "why" steps of your clients' workouts. The better you can communicate this to them, the better their compliance will be. Just think back when you were a kid and your mom asked you to do something (the what). For most of us, our first question (even if not vocalized) was "why?"

This will become second nature as you get more comfortable training people. But until then, simply use the following script as an example:

"Amber, we are going to do a <u>scapular retraction</u> which focuses on the <u>rhomboids</u>. These are the muscles <u>between your shoulder blades and are essential for good posture</u>. When we did your assessment, we talked about <u>the slight rounding in your shoulders and upper back</u>. This exercise will help us correct that issue."

Our clients are intelligent human beings, and they are almost always busy. It is natural for them to want to know why they are doing something and to want to maximize their time with you. I have heard trainers instruct clients with statements, such as "because I'm the trainer" or "this is just the way it's done." I would venture a guess and say those trainers have no clue why they are doing the exercise either.

When programming for your client, research what you are doing and determine why you are doing it. If it is simply to fill time, you may need to shorten their work out time. Why train longer if you can train smarter? And don't let money be an issue here. Charge by the workout, not by the hour. If you are charging $75 for an hour workout but some clients can get the same benefit in half that time, why would you charge less? They are still getting a $75 benefit, right? I was so afraid to try this with my clients but when I did, they were more than happy to be in and out in less time with the same positive results…and at the same price.

Tip Three:
Demonstrate

When you demonstrate the exercise for your clients, they are utilizing their visual learning style. It is very tempting to skip this part of the process. Don't! It is the perfect time to show common form mistakes, such as not retracting and depressing the shoulder girdle before a row (if you don't know why this is essential – stop reading right now and figure it out!).

I find that during the demonstration is when the client is most likely to ask questions about the movement that is unclear to them. Now is a safer time to clarify the movement than when they are actually beginning the movement.

I have observed trainers who apparently just picked an exercise out of a magazine or online and haven't actually tried the exercise. You can imagine how embarrassing it is when they can't remember how to demonstrate the exercise or the exercise doesn't work like they thought it would. Practice all exercises you plan to use and analyze them for safety and efficiency. Just because it is new or different doesn't necessarily make it a great choice.

Tip Four:
Coach

Coaching is the step that engages their kinetic learning style. This is when they are actually doing the exercise. Throughout the exercise you want to give feedback. However, be sensitive to how much they want you to talk to them. Some people need to find their focus and will not be able to get the desired intensity if you interrupt them. Keep your feedback short and sweet with a singular purpose.

Examples of feedback are…

"Turn your toes out a little."

"Lift your chest."

"Excellent! Perfect form!"

"Keep breathing."

A great question while you are coaching is, "where are you feeling this?" You will be amazed where people feel certain exercises. People can be so disconnected from themselves physically.

It can be amusing. I once asked a client where she felt a tricep kickback. Her response was "in my boobs?" I thought I would roll on the floor! You may have to start all over with telling and showing.

To facilitate neuromuscular communication, touch the body part the client is working. This will be crucial for neuromuscular diseases such as multiple sclerosis. And they may have to repeat the exercise several times before they start to feel the correct muscle. (Remember to ask permission before you touch and only touch lightly with your fingertips. This will help protect you legally.)

Also, get on your client's level. If they are on the floor, you should be as well. Never stand over your client. Try to stay eye level with them at all times. This does two things. It shows respect to your client and it allows you to see more clearly how they are doing, allowing you to coach more effectively.

Tip Five:
Evaluate

Now you evaluate what they just did. Make notes on form, weight, reps, complaints, and modifications.

For example, if Mark started out trying a squat but could not maintain proper form, you would modify. If he is quad dominant, put a small lift under his heels. Ninety-nine percent of the time, that small move will correct the problem. If he still can't perfect the form, you may need for him to simply do chair stands and instruct him on how to engage the glutes. Write these things down. Once you are really busy with clients, you may not remember what modifications you made.

The word "personal" in personal training is not a suggestion. It is essential to constantly evaluate and modify your client's progress and workout. One of the things my clients consistently say about me is that I am always adjusting things for their benefit. I have several clients who came to me from larger gyms because they weren't getting the "personal" training they were expecting.

Chapter 5:
Attention!

"Give whatever you are doing
and whoever you are with
the gift of your attention."

Jim Rohn

The Addictive Personal Trainer

Tip One:
Greet them with excitement

The way you greet your client as they enter the door sets the stage for the whole session. I am so fascinated by human behavior that I have experimented with this quite a bit.

There is a major difference in how your client's workout will go if you greet them with an energetic smile, laugh, and/or hug versus a cool smile or a tired or rushed look. In this career field, you are paid to be "on." If you are having a bad day, you may just have to fake it.

Sometimes if I have had a few "EGR" (Extra Grace Required) clients I tell myself, "Fake it 'til you feel it" (Or at least until they all go home and I can scream!) The care and love you show them will not return void. It will most definitely return seven-fold.

One year after opening a new fitness studio, I was diagnosed with an aggressive form of breast cancer. The chemo made me incredibly sick. But I had no choice but to work. My options were to work or lose my business. I wasn't about to lose my business, so I worked.

My clients were beyond amazing! As I worked with clients back to back all day, they set up a system for me. During their warm-up, I would lie down and rest. Then I would get up and train them for 50 minutes. The next person would come in and point to the massage table. I would obediently lie down while they warmed-up and then get up and train them. I even had a client hold my head while I threw up. Yeah, she even paid me for that session. I have the most unbelievable clients who have become some of my best friends over the years.

Invest in them. I promise they will return the favor!

Tip Two:
Take good notes

Keeping good notes benefits you in several ways. It can help keep you protected should someone sue you. It gives a roadmap for another trainer should you need to use a substitute. If you have a manager who oversees what you do, she will appreciate the effort you take to be concise. And it will make your job easier because you won't have to rely on memory for modifications nor will you have to reinvent the wheel anytime changes need to be made to the client's workout.

I note everything. Use codes so you aren't writing a book every time. If we modified a workout for illness, pain, or injury, I make a note. If the client fell at home and reports a sore rib, I make a note. If the client complains of dizziness during our workout and I stopped the workout and suggested a doctor's visit, I make a note! If the client has been out due to any reason and has returned, I make a note. If I know I will be absent, I leave notes for my substitute. You get the picture. In this case, more is always better.

Tip Three:
Eliminate distractions

I have a sign on my studio door that simply says, "By appointment only" and lists my phone number. I keep the door locked.

People often call wanting to "stop by" to meet me, see the studio, or ask a couple of questions. I make it policy to not allow this to happen. When someone is paying me to be their "personal" trainer, they are not happy about sharing that time with anyone else.

Obviously, distractions are a part of life sometimes and I never know the exact time the facility maintenance guy or the water delivery guy will show up. But even then, I respond quickly and efficiently and my client has no doubt where my allegiance lies.

When you don't allow distractions to sidetrack you, it will be easy to start on time and end on time. In my studio, if the client is late, I still end on time.

If the client is early, they wait. Occasionally a client will attempt to get a little extra time before or after their scheduled time. Keep strict boundaries with this. It can get chaotic and overwhelming and it is not fair to you or the client upon whose time they are infringing.

They will respect you more when they know and understand the boundaries you set because no one will be interfering with their time either.

Lastly, stay off your phone. This really should go without saying. But unfortunately, I have clients who say their former trainer texted the whole time they were working out. Seriously? Unbelievable. Enough said on that one!

Tip Four:
Ask about their day/week

People can be very attention-starved. When they have someone who will listen to them and ask them about their life, they will usually respond positively. You must be certain that you are being genuine — they will sense it right away if you are not. They will also ask about your life. It is okay to share something; but keep it brief and turn the conversation back to the client. Once again, this is their time.

Your conversation will affect their workout. If the conversation is negative, there will be a negative effect. I have experimented with this many times. If something bad happened and you or your client discuss what you heard about it on the news, you will notice the client will be weaker, less motivated, and have less stamina. He also will leave feeling less than optimally.

I have one exception to this tip. If a client comes in with a really heavy heart I will probe to see how I can best support them. If you allow her to take the lead, the solution will appear. I have had clients who just needed to work out hard without anyone saying a word and I have had clients who wanted to talk, cry, and/or pray throughout their workout time. It's their time; allow them to spend it how it will best help them walk out your door feeling better.

Conversely, a positive conversation will ignite your client's soul! Read up on good things happening in our world. I use this to jumpstart positive conversations as well as to deter any conversations that start out negatively. You also need to keep yourself in a positive place. If you need a health coach or accountability partner to help you be a more positive force in your clients' lives, then do it! You will gain so much and so will your client.

Tip Five:
Let them know that you enjoy them

As your client is leaving, mention when you will see them again. If there is something you want them to do for their health, remind them of it and that you will want a full report at their next visit. If they are going out of town, tell them you will miss them and can't wait to hear all about their trip. I have clients send pictures, emails, and texts to me while they are out of town. I LOVE that! Yes, it takes time to respond to them, but it is all about building relationships.

Take notes about things you've discussed or events that are happening in your clients' lives. When you ask her how Rover made out with his surgery on Friday, you will win her heart. Who else will remember her dog had surgery? Her friends and family may not have even remembered. If his son is having a birthday party over the weekend, make a note so you will re-member to ask about it on Monday

It is important that this is genuine, so just do what is comfortable for you. I probably go a little overboard because that is just my personality. It's certainly OK to set boundaries as to how involved you want to be in your clients' lives. And I can tell you from experience, the more clients you have, the harder it is to keep up with it. You may need an assistant — even a virtual as-sistant — who is in charge of sending birthday greetings to your clients. Or you may choose to only wish them a happy birthday whatever day they are with you that is closest to their birthday. It's your decision. Do as little or as much as you want, but do something that lets them know they are important to you.

Also if they are out for surgeries or long illnesses, send something to their home. This is a personal touch that is often overlooked in the age of texts and emails. I usually send fruit from Edible Arrangements. They make beautiful creations and it tastes great. My clients always love it.

Chapter 6:
Trust Me!

"To be trusted
is a greater compliment
than being loved."

George MacDonald

Tip One:
Keep what is said in private, private

As a personal trainer, you will become privy to a lot of private information about your clients. Not only will you be gathering medical information, your clients may use their workout time to vent frustrations. These frustrations will often surround primary foods — relationships, career, physical activity, and spirituality. It is imperative that you hold any information they give you in strict confidence.

This is a great opportunity to gain the trust of your client while building a supportive relationship. True health is more than their physical body. The mental, emotional, social, and spiritual aspects all need to be in balance. The more balanced the client's entire life, the happier and healthier they will be. And the more addictive you become.

Tip Two:
Do what you say you will do

A good name is more desirable than great riches; to be esteemed is better than silver or gold. (Proverbs 22:1). Your reputation is everything. It is much easier to maintain a good reputation than to repair a damaged one.

If your client — or potential client — contacts you, make it a policy to return the contact within 24 hours. If you don't have time to address the issue in that time period, send a message to let them know you will get back to them within a set time. Then make sure you do. Integrity is an often-missed character trait in our society. Portray integrity at all times.

If you have agreed to meet a client at 7 a.m., be there early enough to be ready and waiting for the client at 7 sharp. If you have told your client you will email something to them, send it within 24 hours. If you have promised to get them into that bikini by June 1, you better be able to deliver! Remember when making promises, they are with you for a very short time. You cannot control what they are doing the rest of the time.

If you mess up — and you will — be willing to admit fault, apologize, and move on. Once you have done your part to make things right, the ball is in the client's court. You will win most over with your humility and inner strength. However, some may dump you. Don't dwell on it. A mistake is a great learning experience; it is only a failure if you fail to learn something from it.

Tip Three:
Offer accountability

This goes both ways. Your client is accountable to you but you are also accountable to your client. This requires some discernment on your part.

Your clients are accountable to you in many ways. You will help them set and reach goals. In order to reach them, several things may need to be in place. For example, if your clients want to strength train with you twice a week and do cardio at their local gym the other five days, you may need to have them write down in their calendars the exact times they will go to the gym. If clients need nutritional or lifestyle support, you may have to provide them with email or phone support throughout the week. Set boundaries around this support. Times and days should be agreed upon from the beginning, and your time should be compensated. If you charge a sufficient hourly rate and want to include a 15-minute phone chat or a couple of email chats per week, that is OK. Just don't shortchange yourself. You are offering a valuable service, and people will take it more seriously when they are paying for it.

You also are accountable to your client. You must be willing to listen to them and trust them enough to allow them to maintain a lead role in their care. Have the strength of character to accept criticism from them and to learn from it. I do not believe "the customer is always right" because no one is always right. So this is where the discernment comes in. If you have one client who always complains about something and you have tried to accommodate them to no avail, it may be time to recommend they think about finding a new trainer. Sometimes your sanity is worth more than the money they are paying you. But even in this situation, remember to be respectful in your words and actions toward them.

The Addictive Personal Trainer

Tip Four:
Be strong

Strength is multi-faceted. For your client to trust you as a trainer, you must be physically strong, obviously. But you must also be professionally strong. Are you professionally resilient and courageous? Do you take criticism well? Are you able to make tough decisions? Do you bounce back from challenges? Are you tough enough to stay strong when things go wrong?

In order to help impact your clients positively, you must be strong enough to provide support and assistance to them without allowing your own life to interfere. Your client's workout time is your primary concern, regardless of what else is going on in the gym. There can be a lot of drama among trainers and staff and the client will sense it even if they don't know exactly what is happening. It is your job to protect them from this pettiness. You want to make the client feel like he is the only person in the place.

Being strong professionally will also keep you in a positive mindset, which will make you a better trainer, employee, and person. A few tips for being strong professionally are:

■ Support good ideas — even if they aren't your own
■ If you know you are right, listen as if you are wrong
■ Provide assistance and support to others in achieving their goals
■ Admit what you don't know
■ Be responsive to your boss' priorities and your team's needs
■ Don't participate in gossip or negative talk

- When in the presence of clients or potential clients, be a stand-out — smile, laugh, greet, assist — allow only positive energy to flow from you
- Be a good example to everyone there
- Always remember that every decision you make will impact your future, so decide carefully

Tip Five:
Be real — not the stereotypical trainer

The stereotypical trainer has many faces depending on the client's perceptions about the industry and their personal experiences in the industry. When I first started out in the fitness field, I was into bodybuilding. Naturally, I wanted to maximize muscle and minimize fat. My eating regimen was super strict and my mind was obsessed with analyzing every calorie I consumed and every calorie I burned (oh, and of course how I looked in a mirror).

This lifestyle is perfect for some people, and I give great kudos to them. However, what I can now tell you about that time is that I had very few friends and very few clients. And the interesting part is that I really didn't even notice since my entire existence was all about me.

I had never experienced a weight problem so I had no compassion for anyone who — in my opinion — "chose" to be fat. I was a typical "I work hard for this body and if you do what I do, you will look like me" trainer. The problem? Well for starters, not everyone wants to be obsessed with what they eat and how much they work out, not to mention that is not a healthy or a particularly happy life. Secondly, unless they are also into bodybuilding, they may be too intimidated by the fact that you look like one.

My clientele exploded in early 1992. I was the heaviest I had been since I started working at that gym. People began flocking to my classes and my personal training schedule was full. (I will say that my male clientele stayed consistent throughout, so for me this was more about how women feel about female trainers.)

I couldn't figure it out, so I started asking people what was drawing them to my sessions. The answers I got from women were that I looked more normal and they felt they could attain the physique I had. What no one knew at the time was that I was five months pregnant. I gained 18 pounds during my pregnancy and was the busiest I had ever been in the gym. After the pregnancy, I decided I wanted to stay at a more "normal" weight. I was happier and able to focus my energy on other people, not just myself.

Another thing I hear is that some trainers simply push too hard. If your client is always sore, you may be pushing them too hard. Is it really necessary to hurry them into results that you can ease them into with less pain? I encourage you to rethink what health, wellness, and fitness should look like. There are certainly exceptions. Some people love this chronic soreness but you must remember, that is not true for everyone.

Another way to "be real" is simply to allow the client into your world. This shouldn't be a "tell-all" about your life, but real people like to work with other real people. If you have a soft spot for chocolate cake and are easily tempted, share that at an opportune time when your client has fallen into temptation. It's okay for them to know you have temptations, and it is OK for them to know you indulge at times. My clients know that I plan any trip past Krispy Kreme Doughnuts during times that they do not have on the "HOT AND NOW" sign. And if I must go past there during that time, I do one of two things: I either position myself in traffic so I am the farthest lane away from Krispy Kreme or I decide I'm going in. However, they also know I may do this two or three times a year, not two or three times a week.

Think about people you admire. Are they perfect or can you relate to them? I love people who know they aren't perfect, who don't try to be perfect, and especially, who don't expect me to be perfect! I have perfectionist tendencies and I have worked very hard to be free from that bondage. If you have those tendencies — and many people in our field do — learn to love yourself and give yourself freedom to fail. You will be a better trainer and a much happier person.

Chapter 7: Encourage, encourage, encourage ... oh, and did I say, encourage?

"A good coach will make his players
see what they can be
rather than what they are."

Ara Parasheghian

Tip One:
Realize everyone needs encouragement

According to a research experiment led by Lysann Damisch of the University of Cologne in Germany, a dexterity task that normally took more than five minutes was accomplished on average in just over three minutes if participants received a good luck message before they started. There are many opinions about how many positive comments it takes to offset a negative one. I have seen ratios go from 2:1 to 9:1. I believe they are all credible depending on the mindset of the person who is receiving the comments.

Someone who is generally positive and feels good about themselves probably does OK with a closer ratio. Others who have been terribly hurt psychologically, who haven't really found their passion in life, or who are simply missing the "happy gene" — yes, researchers really have discovered a "happy gene"— may need a ratio closer to 9:1. When dealing with your clients, it is really pretty easy to determine their encouragement needs simply by listening to them. And it is so easy to do. Think of how little effort it takes to tell someone they just maintained perfect form on an exercise, or that you can really see progress in a specific area they have been working to improve. Of course, you must be sincere; but I can always find something positive to say to anyone, even my EGRs I spoke of earlier. If you missed that comment, EGR stands for "Extra Grace Required."

BONUS TIP: Dr. Gary Chapman, a pastor, speaker, and author who speaks extensively throughout the U.S. and internationally on marriage, family, and relationships teaches that everyone has a "love language" that dictates how they will feel and receive love. Encouragement is one of them. The others are Quality Time, Physical Touch and Closeness, Acts of Service, and Gifts. I love figuring out how my clients feel loved. When you speak to people, it is your natural tendency to speak in your own love language. But if it is not the receiver's love language, it is like hearing a foreign language. It won't make them feel loved. Learn more about love languages (see Appendix). It has the power to change every relationship in your life.

Tip Two:
Make the client want to be around you

When you think about magnetic personalities, what comes to mind? Who comes to mind? What makes them magnetic? Do you encompass any of the qualities you just envisioned?

Why do you think you would make a good personal trainer? Make a list right now on the side of the page. Would you hire yourself? Would your family and friends hire someone based on what you wrote? Ask them.

Sometimes it is hard to determine what qualities we have that people want in a trainer. I asked myself that once and sat twiddling my thumbs. So I asked my friends, family, and clients what made me a good trainer. Talk about encouragement! I would not have recognized myself if these qualities had been written down without my name attached. I had to ask follow-up questions to some people because I had no idea how they came up with certain qualities they saw in me. This little exercise gave me insight into areas where I wanted to see growth as well as areas I felt might need downplaying. And overall, it gave me tons of encouragement.

Two characteristics that I look for when hiring trainers to work in my studio are confidence and empathy. These two words hold a plethora of qualities that result in being a successful personal trainer.

Confidence is the state of feeling certain about the truth of something. I look for a candidate who is certain about their ability to change and improve the lives of others through proven methods that produce proven results. How does this look in a personal trainer? If they approach clients with confidence, they will be bold, energetic, and enthusiastic. They will make proper eye contact, ask the right questions, produce the right plan, and leave the client knowing they are in good hands. This is NOT arrogance. Arrogance tries to impress others while confidence doesn't care whether others are impressed or not. Arrogance is condescending. Confidence is respectful. Arrogance blames others. Confidence accepts fault. Arrogance "one-ups" everybody while confidence doesn't need to brag because the accomplishments do it for them. Arrogance has an answer for everything while confidence has the guts to say, "I don't know, but I will find out."

So ask yourself, "Am I arrogant or confident?" No one finds arrogance addictive. Just sayin'…

Empathy is understanding and entering into another's feelings. This is not sympathy or feeling sorry for someone. I want a trainer who truly understands where people are in their relationships, careers, physical activities, spirituality, and nutrition. People generally become more empathetic as they get older and have experienced more in their lives.

Some people are just born with an ability to empathize with others. They are sometimes referred to as empaths. Empaths are people who don't "read" the future, but "read" the people. They're often problem-solvers, thinkers, and students of many things. As far as empaths are concerned, where there is a problem, there is an answer.

Of course a trainer doesn't have to be an empath to show empathy for their clientele. As a trainer learns to show empathy, the clientele will have no problems opening up and allowing the trainer access into parts of their lives that are just as important as their workouts. The goal must be for healthy, holistic people, not just people who can complete an impressive workout.

The Addictive Personal Trainer

Tip Three:
Celebrate the small victories

Small victories become great ones. Never underestimate the power of baby steps. A Chinese proverb that I have always loved states, "The journey of a thousand miles begins with a single step."

Life in general can be so discouraging for people. I absolutely agree with Bill Gates when he said, "The world won't care about your self-esteem. The world will expect you to accomplish something BEFORE you feel good about yourself." I have heard a lot of people take great issue with this statement. But please notice he said "something" not "something big." If it weren't for people accomplishing the little things in life, no one would be able to accomplish the big things. Bill Gates was aware of this. Look at all the people that helped him accomplish what he did.

I believe, as personal trainers, we can help people feel good about themselves with very little effort. My clients get pumped anytime they see their times get better, their muscles get stronger, their pants get looser! And many times these are small changes. But just you watch, these small changes turn into lifelong habits that turn into monumental health and happiness victories, often not only for your clients, but for their families, friends, and co-workers.

I give stickers. Not all the time so they become routine, but when someone does especially well or has accomplished a goal. It is funny how people still love getting a sticker from the "teacher." It is an inexpensive way to help celebrate those small victories.

Tip Four:
Laugh A LOT

"Hearty laughter is a good way to jog internally without having to go outdoors. " Norman Cousins

Laughter will help you bond with your clients, help them relax, and make them want to come back for more laugh-therapy. Laughter is a sign of joy and cheerfulness. Even the Bible says in Proverbs 17:22, "A joyful heart is good medicine, but a crushed spirit dries up the bones."

Do you train people with osteoporosis? Check in on their spirit. A crushed spirit is simply a discouraged spirit, a spirit that feels unloved, anxious, depressed. As a trainer, you can be a catalyst for the joy they — and their bones — so badly need.

. Physically, laughter also:
Lowers blood pressure
Increases heart rate and blood flow
Increases pain tolerance. People with chronic pain issues, especially fibromyalgia — can benefit.
Provides a workout to the muscles of the diaphragm and to the abdominal, respiratory, facial, leg, and back muscles
Improves alertness, creativity, and memory
Reduces stress hormones such as cortisol and adrenaline (Research shows that laughter can serve to reduce stress long after a bout of laughter has ended.)
Increases the response of tumor-killing and disease-killing cells such as gamma-interferon and T-cells and helps the body defend against respiratory infections — even reducing the fre-

quency of colds — by increasing immunoglobulin in the saliva. Mentally, laugh or humor therapy is a growing trend. Laughter is cathartic. It serves as a release mechanism for negative emotions such as anger, sadness and fear. Laughter also incites relaxation and inhibits the fight-or-flight response. Laughter is useful for decreasing interpersonal tension and helps train people to have control over emotional responses.

You can suggest laughter meditation to your client. Have your client stretch every muscle in her body like a cat. Sit still for a few moments and then start laughing. It may be necessary to force laughter a little at the beginning. Some techniques for starting a laugh include saying, 'Ha, Ha, Ha,' or 'Ho, Ho, Ho,' to get the laughter energy moving. Allow for spontaneous laughter to arise. Most likely, the attempt itself will be silly enough to incite natural laughter. Try it for five minutes. If natural laughter does not occur, simply continue to practice each day. Sometimes it is easier with another person because you will both feel so silly about it.

Tip Five:
Help them be positive

A great question to ask your client is "What is new and good with you today?" You may be surprised how many people will not be able to answer that question. And the ones who do often give fact-based answers that seem very proper and contrived. As a society we aren't supposed to share the positives are we? Won't that make us seem conceited? Or insensitive to the woes of the world?

But you can train your clients to focus on the positives that happen all day long but get overlooked. Once they realize you are going to be asking this question, they will start remembering things to share. And it is beautiful. My clients often come through the door smiling ear to ear and proclaiming something good that has happened to them. I love it. Can you imagine how much better their workout will be? It is a totally different experience for them...and for the trainer, too!

Some clients will continue to want the attention they get from sharing all the negatives. I'm not saying you shouldn't be there to support the negative as well; but just don't allow them to wallow in it. I once had an evaluation with a client who kept talking about wanting to lose weight. I asked her if she was mad about it yet. She said no, that she was just upset. I politely said I couldn't help her until she got mad about it. Staying upset is staying in the self-pity mode. People don't make positive changes there. She was shocked, hired me, got mad, changed her life, and became incredibly happy. That, my friends, is what I call success!

I have also had good luck with gratitude journals. If I notice someone just can't seem to recall any positives unless prompted, I give them a small journal that they can keep in their car or purse. When good things happen, they record it in the journal. When they come in for their warm-up, we celebrate what they have written. It starts their workout off on the right foot.

Guide your clients to also "pay-it-forward" by encouraging others in their lives to focus on positivity and gratitude. I have seen this bring healing and closeness into families and friendships.

As your client shares how they have helped others, their own light will begin to shine even brighter.

And as their light shines brighter, so will yours.

Chapter 8:
Learn More,
Earn More

"Get over the idea
that only children should spend
their time in study.
Be a student so long as you
still have something to learn,
and this will mean all your life."

Henry L. Doherty

Tip One:
Stay up to date on research and trends

In the fitness/wellness field, knowledge is most definitely power. The more you can comprehensively help your clients, the more they will rely on you. It is imperative that you stay up to date on research and trends. Your client reads them daily in all sorts of places. I love to engage them mentally in the process of analyzing what they are reading. This is especially true with nutrition. If you can teach them how to properly analyze the research — specifically how to research WHO did the research, you will have blessed them with a very valuable skill. For example, be leery of anyone who has a financial interest in the results of the research.

There are lots of great resources out there to help you stay current on research and trends. Check into the World Instructor Training Schools, the American Council on Exercise, IDEA Health and Fitness Association, the American College of Sports Medicine, the National Strength and Conditioning Association, On Fitness magazine, and Men's Health.

It's lots of fun to go to workshops. I always pick places that I want to visit and then choose a workshop in that area. That way my "vacation" is tax-deductible. Plus, it is a great networking opportunity to meet other trainers and exchange ideas. Don't be one of those trainers who think the fitness world begins and ends with them. Learn from everyone.

Another way to stay current is through online courses. They are easy and available when you are. Workshops and online courses will supply you with the proper continuing education credits to maintain your certification.

Trends can be fun and at the same time aggravating. If there is a simple trend that your client thinks they would love and you can safely accommodate, do it. It probably won't last long; but it lets them know you are listening to them. Never get so cocky with what you do that you can't be open to new ideas. Boredom is a main reason for losing clients. So if a trend will keep them interested, it's an easy way to keep them happy and to nurture their addiction to you.

The Addictive Personal Trainer

Tip Two:
Become the go-to expert

When people first started telling me I needed a target market, I didn't want to listen. And when they began constantly saying it's better to be "a big fish in a small pond than a small fish in a big pond" I just rolled my eyes at the stupid cliché. Well, now I use the same stupid cliché.

There are lots of people with very different health and fitness goals. If you can become the expert in a certain area, your business will actually grow.

I know it sounds counter-intuitive. It seems like if you just take anyone you would have more opportunity to be in demand. However, if you were to choose a handyman who did everything pretty well or a painter who did one thing amazingly well for the same price, who would you hire to paint your living room?

How do you determine a target market? Purpose follows passion.

Figure out your ultimate passion. If your passion is to work with disabled children, then set your goals and experiences up to prepare for that. Why waste time getting experience with the general population if disabled children are your passion?

Have you always had a heart for wounded veterans? Research where to go to get the experience needed to work with them and make contacts to get into those jobs.

With social networking, meet-up groups, and workshop opportunities, your possibilities are totally endless. Grab your passion by the horns and make your dreams come true!

Tip Three:
Learn about nutrition

Michael Pollan: "Eat food. Not too much. Mostly plants."

There are few subjects more frustrating and controversial than nutrition. Research from the American Society for Clinical Nutrition determined that most medical schools are not providing adequate nutrition instruction. Furthermore, the study found that most of the instruction received is within other subjects such as biochemistry or physiology and not in a format designed specifically for nutrition curriculum.

As an entry-level personal trainer you must be careful not to "prescribe" diets. It is out of your scope of practice. However, ask any fitness professional or nutrition expert and you will hear that diet is 70 to 90 percent responsible for transforming and improving body and health. See the dilemma? You have a few options. You could go back to college and get a degree in nutrition or dietetics (the most time-consuming option), follow the government guidelines for nutrition (my least favorite option), or sign up for my mentoring program at www.rhondakhuff. com where you will learn enough basics to give your clients the jumpstart they need to achieve great health.

In the meantime, here is an acronym that I developed to help people remember how to eat:

Just eat real
F.O.O.D™ !

Free of unpronouncables

Original in form

Organic when possible

Dense in nutrients

Free of unpronounceables: The ingredient list is more important than the "Nutrition Facts" label. If you can't pronounce it, don't eat it. Also, as a general rule, if there are more than five ingredients, don't bother trying to pronounce it, just put it back on the shelf.

Original in form: A chicken breast should look like a breast, not a dinosaur. Choose whole fruits instead of fruits that have been changed from the original form. For example, an apple is better than applesauce, which is better than apple juice, which is better than apple pie. Michael Pollan puts it this way, "Don't eat anything your great-great-grandmother wouldn't recognize as food."

Organic when possible: I know, I know, "It's too expensive to eat organic." Well guess what, it's even more expensive to get chemo later to kill the cancer the pesticides cause. It has always baffled me that God created us to be the smartest of all creation and yet we eat food that other animals won't touch. Does that even make sense? If your clients stop buying crap and stop eating between meals they can easily afford the organic and save on medical bills in the process. (Yes, I said stop eating between meals. Unless you are an elite athlete, you should only be eating three times per day. The United States of America is the only country that eats more than this!) Also, refer them to www.ewg.org to read the "Shopper's Guide to Pesticides" which will empower them to make informed choices.

Dense in nutrients: The more the better. An easy method is Dr. David Katz' Nuval Nutritional Scoring System (www.nuval.com). Using the "original form" apple example from above, an apple has a Nuval

Score of 96 and applesauce has a Nuval Score of 4. Broccoli and blueberries both have Nuval Scores of 100! Another informative nutrient site is www.whfoods.com/foodstoc.php.

Supplementation is also an extremely confusing topic. When dealing with supplements, a little knowledge is a dangerous thing. Even protein powders are usually full of trash that we should not have in our bodies. So tread carefully. Many supplements are not needed if your client is eating real food. Vitamins and minerals that have been extracted from a whole food is missing an important element: synergy! It is the synergistic combination of the thousands of healthy nutrients found in vegetables, fruit, whole grains, beans, peas, nuts, and seeds working together that protect our health. The supplements that some of your clients may need are

B12 (if they eat little or no animal protein)

D which is technically a hormone and not a vitamin because it is produced in the body. If you live north of 37 degrees latitude, which would be approximately a line drawn horizontally connecting Norfolk, VA, to San Francisco, CA, sunlight is not sufficient to create Vitamin D in your skin in the winter months, even if you are sitting in the sun in a bathing suit on a warm January day. The further you live from the equator, the longer exposure you need to the sun in order to generate vitamin D. Since Vitamin D is fat-soluble, I ask my clients to have their level checked by their doctor before they start taking it. They need to ask for a 25-hydroxy vitamin D test.

Omega-3 We associate omega-3 fatty acids with fish, but fish get them from green plants, specifically algae. Plant leaves produce these essential fatty acids (they are called "essential" because our bodies can't produce them on their own) as part of photosynthesis. Seeds contain more of another essential fatty acid: omega-6. Omega-3s and Omega-6s perform totally different functions. Omega-3s play an important role in neurological development and processing, the permeability of cell walls, the metabolism of glucose, and the calming of inflammation. Omega-6s are involved in fat storage (which is what they do for the plant), the rigidity of cell walls, clotting, and the inflammation response. Since they compete with each other for the attention of important enzymes, the ratio between Omega-3s and Omega-6s may matter more than the absolute quantity of either fat. Thus too much Omega-6 may be just as much a problem as too little Omega-3. Anyone eating a Western diet is unfortunately getting more Omega-6s due to less consumption of leafy greens and more consumption of factory-farmed meats, polyunsaturated vegetable oils, and hydrogenated oils. The typical Western diet has an Omega-6 to Omega-3 ratio of more than 10:1, some estimate it is closer to 20:1. The maximum safe ratio is considered to be 4:1; but before the turn of the 19th century, the ratio was closer to 1:1.

Tip Four:
Learn life/health coaching

Dr. Oz recently completed a survey asking people what their top three complaints were about their doctor. The No. 3 complaint was "doing too many tests." The No. 2 and No. 1 complaints respectively were: "doesn't listen to me" and "rushes me through the visit." The bad news is: This trend is expected to continue. The good news is: This trend is expected to continue. The rise of life/health coaching is concurrent with the decline of satisfying doctor/patient relationships. Life/health coaching is a perfect complement to personal training. It creates what I call the perfect triangle – exercise, nutrition, and lifestyle, each in perfect balance with the others.

I researched life/health coaching programs for over five years before choosing the Institute for Integrative Nutrition. I learned more than I ever thought imaginable. Joshua Rosenthall, the institute's founder, has absolutely covered all the bases in his Health Coach Training Program. His unique formula of bioindividuality, primary foods, deconstructing cravings, and crowding out the bad stuff ensures renowned success for the clients. Plus we are taught by the world's foremost experts in nutrition and wellness like Dr. Andrew Weil, Dr. Arthur Agatston, Dr. Mark Hyman, Dr. David Katz, Deepak Chopra, David Wolfe, Geneen Roth, and so many more amazing people!

Check out their free 342 page nutrition book on my website, www.rhondakhuff.com!

Tip Five:
Surround yourself with experts

Never discount how much you can learn from other people. If you will keep an open mind about the wellness field, you can learn from anyone, including your clients. Personal training clients are always reading and listening to fitness information. Granted, some of it is crap, but that is okay. Sometimes they can give you little nuggets to hold on to which just makes you an even better trainer.

And when you sincerely listen to what they have to say, you make them feel important. That's a great way to retain clients.

If you know people who are more successful than yourself, see if they are willing to mentor you. Most fitness/wellness professionals want to help as many people as possible, and sometimes they are willing to share their ideas with you so you can help carry the torch successfully.

If you are the type of person who wants to be the know-it-all about our field, your growth potential will fall exponentially. Don't allow yourself to be ego-driven about what you know, or think you know.

There is always so much new research out there that it is absolutely impossible to know everything.

The more we help each other, the more we can help those who need us most.

I love this poem (author unknown)…

"Today I choose to live by choice,
not by chance;
To make changes, not excuses.
To be motivated, not manipulated.
To be useful, not used.
To excel, not compete.
I choose self-esteem, not self-pity.
I choose to listen to my inner voice,
not the random opinion of others."

Our reach is colossal, our impact, crucial.

You have the skills.
You know enough.
Keep learning as a trainer.
Keep growing as a person.

Now, go! Get out there and make a difference.

People need a new addiction.
And that addiction is YOU!

"Don't wait until everything is just right. It will never be perfect. There will always be challenges, obstacles and less than perfect conditions. So what. Get started now. With each step you take, you will grow stronger and stronger, more and more skilled, more and more self-confident and more and more successful."

Mark Victor Hansen

The Addictive Personal Trainer

Take the Next Step

I mentor a limited number of new personal trainers each year. I provide support in the following areas:

Setting Personal and Professional Goals

Finding and Retaining Clients

Business Development and Marketing

Personal Health Coaching

Simple Health Coaching Strategies to Use with Clients

How to Give Successul Workshops and Lectures

Building Your Own Confidence Level

Nutritional Concepts

Program Design

For information on these programs or to submit questions, go to www.rhondakhuff.com today.

The Addictive Personal Trainer

Appendix

Visit my website at
www.rhondakhuff.com

The World Instructor Training Schools
www.witseducation.com

Institute for Integrative Nutrition
www.bodyinbalance757.com (click on the free book offer)

The Trigger Point Therapy Workbook: Your Self-Treatment
Guide for Pain Relief by Clair Davies
www.amazon.com

IDEA Health & Fitness Association
www.ideafit.com

Gray Cook, Physical Therapist
www.graycook.com

Tom Purvis, Physical Therapist
www.resistancetrainingspecialist.com

The Nuval Food Scoring System
www.nuval.com

Pete Cerqua
90-secondfitness.com

The Addictive Personal Trainer

About the Author

My own fitness journey began as a sophomore in high school. My track coach incorporated weightlifting into our training program, and I was hooked. It was amazing! I felt so empowered – like I could do anything! I began looking forward to weight training much more than track practice itself! Shortly after graduating, I joined a gym and began bodybuilding with one of the trainers at the gym. It was so exhilarating for me, giving me a feeling of power and accomplishment that I carried with me through the rest of the day.

At 19, I signed up to take an aerobics class for PE credit in college (at the time I was an accounting major). There I found another interest and started teaching some of their aerobics classes the very next semester. After my first year of school, I switched majors, knowing I wanted to work in fitness. I decided to pursue a Bachelor of Science degree in Fitness/Wellness with a concentration in post-rehab and injury prevention.

Since that time, I have worked with the Air Force, athletes, youth and children, post-rehab patients, weight-loss clients, special populations, geriatrics and people looking for general wellbeing. I do numerous lectures on health and fitness, own a successful personal training and health coaching business, teach personal training classes, and mentor new trainers.

One thing has always remained the same: It's all about the client – what the client wants, needs, feels, loves, and hates. When you become sincerely client-focused, everyone wins.

You achieve success and the client achieves far more than they expected.

The Addictive Personal Trainer

What People are Saying

The very best part of working out with Rhonda is that she tailors the routine individually to each client. She is amazingly knowledgeable and can fine-tune any workout to maximize benefits in specific areas of need. She keeps herself up to date on advancements in her field and I certainly feel that she is always devoted to my overall wellness and fitness. Thanks, Rhonda!!

— Maureen Hutchens

I went to Rhonda 8 years ago with such an unbelievable postural imbalance that I could hardly look forward. I also suffered from a condition called Charcot-Marie-Tooth which prevents you from lifting your toes, which leads to frequent falling. I had tried physical therapy, but there was no real supervision and I did not get any better. Rhonda had the knowledge and provided the one-on-one treatment that I needed and now I walk everywhere and work fulltime. Without Rhonda I know I would be crippled and in a wheelchair.

— Sheila Rubin

I fully endorse Rhonda Greene as my personal life-saver. She always greets me with a big smile and a contagious laugh. Her relentless desire to improve my strength and overall health has resulted in meeting and exceeding goals I never thought achievable. Her dedication and unique methods have made me a better person. Don't hesitate to get your body in balance. Start today.

— Lorrie Brantley

Rhonda, upon the completion of your program, or shall I say the ongoing lifestyle change that I have chosen to pursue for better health and awareness, I am forever indebted. Thinking back over the past six months, I have learned not only about better health habits and nutrition, but my awareness of the two and how they impact me and my family. Every day I make choices of what to eat, how much physical activity I engage in, how I interact with others, and how much stress I allow to enter my life. These choices not only affect me, but my family as well. Your program has changed how I feel about the choices that I make for myself and my family. The integrative nutrition portion of your program is unique in that I was able to concentrate on how different food groups make my body feel throughout the day. Switching to greens and experi-

menting with foods that I had not even heard of was fun and delicious. My two year old loves salads now. The mid-afternoon cravings switched from sugary carbs to raw fruits and vegetables. I no longer feel the need to crash on the couch after work, but instead I have the stamina to clean my house, play with my daughter, and enjoy being with my family. The exercise portion of the program taught me that anytime can be a good time for a workout. I restructured my "routine" day and practiced yoga during my lunch. Every morning has been a wonderful time for stretching and for meditation. I have learned how to relax and enjoy my time instead of being ruled by other people's demands. I have learned how to listen to my body and I know the importance of taking care of myself spiritually and physically. Most importantly is the self-discovery process of your program. Through journaling, I have learned things about my stress and anxiety that I have suppressed for years. I no longer feel the need to bottle up my feelings, but have learned to be more expressive. I share what I have learned with friends and family because I know this program works and has the potential to change other people's lives. With every milestone that I have made, I have become a stronger person. I deal with stress in different ways and I have a new passion for life. Food is no longer a comfort that injures my body, but an enjoyment for nourishment the way God intended. I still feel like I am discovering new things with your

*program and I intend to be an active participant in
my own self-exploration! Thank you for your time and
teaching! My world has changed and I am better for it
thanks to you and your program. You are a wonderful
teacher!!!!*

— **Karla Gentry**

*I can definitely say my life has been changed. I have
acquired the knowledge and motivation I need to be a
healthier, happier me. I am learning to eat healthier
foods and LIKING them, my priorities are clearer and
I am finding blessings in every day. Rhonda has a true
gift for inspiring people and it is evident that she loves
what she does and cares about the whole person. I am
in turn helping my family with what I have learned
and have the tools to create a healthier home. This is a
wonderful program and Rhonda is a wonderful coach!*

— **Michele Brooks**

*Rhonda is one of the nicest people I have ever met.
She shares wonderful tips and explanations for why we
crave certain foods. She is very positive, outgoing, and
exactly what people need. She also has awesome ideas
for de-stressing and making positive changes. During*

my 6 months with Rhonda I have become more asser-
tive in a male-dominated work environment which has
helped me gain their respect. I am eating and loving
lots of new foods. I am sleeping so much better and feel
so healthy. I have become much more positive and fo-
cused on my future and made it into an MBA program!

— **Christa Riley**

My legs were causing me great pain. I would feel like
I was walking on stilts and had to curtail many ac-
tivities. I found Rhonda through a newspaper article.
Thank God for the article and for Rhonda!! Rhonda
worked with me and helped me strengthen my leg mus-
cles so that I could resume activities. I was very afraid
of working out but Rhonda started slowly and stayed
by my side every minute of my time with her, giving
me encouragement and making sure I was doing the
exercises correctly. Rhonda's encouragement, positive
attitude, knowledge, and patience are why I now call
her "my guardian angel."

— **Nancy G**

I have been a client of Rhonda's for 8 years. I used
to have a trainer at a local gym but he often used the

same routines for all his clients and they did not always fit every client – especially not me. It was very discouraging. One of the things I like most about Rhonda's training style is that she really listens to what her clients want to change about their bodies and then she designs an exercise routine based on the client's goals. She constantly tweaks the exercises as needed and she changes the routines every 6-8 weeks so the client doesn't plateau. Rhonda constantly researches exercise and nutrition and incorporates her findings into her sessions, thus assuring the optimum results for her clients.

— Judy P

The Addictive Personal Trainer

www.ingramcontent.com/pod-product-compliance
Lightning Source LLC
Chambersburg PA
CBHW072237290326
41934CB00008BB/1318